GET 30% HAPPIER IN JUST 30 DAYS!

After the global pandemic, Americans are the unhappiest they've been since the Great Depression, and it's causing big problems. Being unhappy is associated with increased stress, fatigue, weight gain, heart disease, premature aging, and a harder (and shorter) life. And it puts a strain on relationships. Depression has tripled, and anxiety and addictions have reached record highs. This is so sad.

But it doesn't have to be this way. You can learn to cultivate happiness even when it seems like the world is crumbling around you. Researchers have spent decades trying to decode happiness, but they have completely missed 7 important aspects. Over the past 30+ years at Amen Clinics, our brain SPECT imaging work (over 180,000 brain scans and growing!) and clinical practice has taught us so much. We have discovered the 7 neuroscience secrets to happiness that no one is talking about but that everyone should be talking about!

In this journal, I will share the 7 neuroscience secrets to happiness as well as 7 questions you need to ask yourself each day. Incorporating them into daily life sparks happiness. I've seen it happen. In 2021, I created a 30-Day Happiness Challenge for which over 32,000 people signed up. After a month, their self-reported happiness scores went up over 30%—and their energy went up 30% too—using the same tools you'll read about here. And they did it in just a few focused minutes a day!

Your 30-day happiness journey starts here, and this daily journal will guide you every joyful step of the way.

Before You Begin

How happy (or unhappy) are you? To track your progress on your happiness journey, you need to know where you're starting. Take the Oxford Happiness Questionnaire at 30DayHappinessChallenge.com to find your happiness score.

How to Use This Journal

Each day, you'll discover a proven strategy to boost your moods based on one or more of the 7 neuroscience secrets. Think of it as your daily dose of happiness! You'll be guided to focus on one specific happiness exercise each day. And to help you make happiness a habit, use the daily journal to answer the 7 questions each and every day.

Are you ready to get happier? Let's get started!

Daniel G. Amen, MD

CONTENTS

DAY 1. LEARN THE 7 SECRETS AND 7 QUESTIONS *(Relates to Secrets 1-7)*

Your happiness journey begins today by becoming familiar with the 7 neuroscience secrets to happiness that most researchers completely ignore but that everyone should be talking about. In addition, take note of the 7 questions you need to ask yourself every day to get happier. These secrets and questions will be explored in greater detail throughout your 30-day journey and more will be revealed in the coming days.

Secret 1: Know your Brain Type.

Question 1: Am I focused on what makes me uniquely happy each day?

Secret 2: Optimize the physical functioning of your brain.

Question 2: Is this good for my brain or bad for it?

Secret 3: Nourish your unique brain.

Question 3: Am I nourishing my unique brain?

Secret 4: Choose foods you love that love you back

Question 4: Do I choose foods today I love that love me back?

Secret 5: Master your mind and gain psychological distance from the noise in your head.

Question 5: Is it true? And what went well today?

Secret 6: Notice what you like about others more than what you don't.

Question 6: Am I reinforcing the behaviors I like or dislike in others today?

Secret 7: Live each day based on your clearly defined values, purpose, and goals.

Question 7: Does it fit? Does my behavior today fit the goals I have for my life?

At Amen Clinics, we have also learned that the 7 secrets of happiness happen in 4 Circles.

- **Biological Circle:** How your physical body and brain function (Secrets 1-4)
- **Psychological Circle:** Developmental issues and how you think (Secret 5)
- **Social Circle:** Social network, life situation, and societal influences (Secret 6)
- **Spiritual Circle:** Your connection to God, the planet, past and future generations, and your deepest sense of meaning and purpose (Secret 7)

Throughout this 30-day journey, you will discover more about the 4 Circles of Happiness. For now, here are a few examples of ways all of the Brain Types can increase happiness in the 4 Circles:

Biological Circle
Exercise targeted to your Brain Type
Physical affection
Gaze into your spouse's eyes
Get a massage
Get 7-8 hours of sleep

Psychological Circle
Start your day with "Today is going to be a great day."
Write down any distressing thoughts
Focus on what you like
Watch a comedy
Write down your 5 happiest life experiences

Social Circle
Call a friend
Eat dinner as a family
Send an appreciation text to someone
Limit screen time
Work on your resume

Spiritual Circle
Pray
Meditate
Volunteer
Be a mentor to someone
Do a random act of kindness

Today's exercise: *Learn the 7 secrets and 7 questions.*

"Happiness is a moral obligation." — *Dennis Prager*

DAY 2. DISCOVER YOUR BRAIN TYPE
(Relates to Secret 1)

What makes you happy depends on your Brain Type. SPECT imaging has helped us identify 5 Primary Brain Types (and a total of 16 types). The chart below introduces you to the main types, the SPECT findings, common attributes, and what makes each type happy or unhappy. Knowing what makes your Brain Type happy helps you create a path to lasting contentment.

Brain Type	SPECT Findings	Attributes	Makes This Type Happy	Makes This Type Unhappy
1. Balanced	Balanced, healthy brain	Flexible, focused, good impulse control, balanced emotions, resilient, normal ups and downs	Healthy relationships, meaningful work, financial security, following the rules, being on time, having fun, holiday traditions	Chaos, excessive risk-taking, running late, missing assignments, being around people who are undependable (or negative or rule breakers)
2. Spontaneous	Frontal lobes don't work hard enough	Spontaneous, risk taking, creative "out of the box" thinker, easily distracted, restless, focused only when interested, tendency for ADD	Trying new things, surprises, brainstorming, starting new projects, scary movies, getting a rise out of people	Boredom, sameness, familiarity, having to sit in one place for too long, deadlines, being told you can't do something, waiting in line
3. Persistent	Frontal lobes work too hard	Persistent, strong-willed, relentless, holds on to hurts, gets stuck on thoughts, notices what's wrong more than what's right, tendency for OCD	Being in charge, being respected, predictable days, sameness, familiarity, keeping traditions, routines, making own decisions	People who don't do what they say, failure, getting told no, being kept waiting, being stymied by higher-ups, having the rules changed

Brain Type	SPECT Findings	Attributes	Makes This Type Happy	Makes This Type Unhappy
4. Sensitive	Emotional center works too hard	Sensitive, feels deeply, struggles with negative thoughts, empathetic, struggles with moods, pessimistic, tendency for depression	Calming music, sense of purpose, deep thoughts, scent of lavender, caring for others, alone time, creative expression, journaling	Negative thoughts, being socially disconnected, regretting the past, setbacks at work, busy traffic, loud noises, scary or violent movies
2. Cautious	Anxiety center works too hard	Prepared, cautious, busy-minded, motivated, reserved, restless, tendency for anxiety disorders	Calm environment, being organized, being early, warm baths, making lists, finishing assignments on time (or early)	Chaotic environment, fears about future, being late, having too much to do, reading or watching distressing news

Today's exercise: *Discover your Brain Type by taking our quiz at* <u>*brainhealthassessment.com*</u>

"Happiness is not one-size-fits-all." — Daniel G. Amen, MD

DAY 3. BRIGHT MINDS
(Relates to Secret 2)

Today is such an important day in your happiness journey. This is the day when you learn that brain health is foundaticnal to happiness. When your brain works right, you work right. When your brain is troubled, for whatever reason, you're much more likely to have trouble in your life and to be unhappy.

At Amen Clinics, we created a mnemonic—a memory device—to help you remember what's good for your brain or bad for it: BRIGHT MINDS. See the chart below to learn more about the 11 risk factors, things that increase your risk, and the Happy Brain Habits that help prevent or treat these risk factors.

BRIGHT MINDS RISK FACTORS & STRATEGIES

Factors	Risks	Happy Brain Habits
B is for Blood Flow Low blood flow is the #1 brain imaging predictor of Alzheimer's disease.	Stroke Hypertension Any form of heart disease Little to no exercise	Get treatment early Start prevention strategies Eat foods such as beets and cayenne pepper Take supplements such as Ginkgo Exercise (30 minutes a day)
R is for Retirement/Aging When you stop learning your brain starts dying.	No new learning In a job that does not require new learning Loneliness Social isolation	Make new learning part of your everyday life Take a class Get involved with your family or church Volunteer to help others
I is for Inflammation Inflammation markers include C-reactive protein and omega-3 index.	Standard American Diet (SAD) filled with fast and processed food Low omega-3 levels High C-reactive protein (CRP) levels	Eat an anti-inflammatory diet Increase dietary omega-3 fatty acids Take supplements, such as fish oil, probiotics, and curcumins
G is for Genetic Vulnerabilities Genetic risk is not a death sentence. It's a wake-up call!	Family history of mental health issues or dementia	If you have a family history of mental health issues or dementia, get serious about brain health as soon as possible Get screened early

Factors	Risks	Happy Brain Habits
H is for Head Trauma/ Concussions If you put the brain in a healing environment, it can get better.	Head injury even without loss of consciousness	Protect your head Wear a helmet when biking, skiing, etc. Refrain from contact sports Wear your seat belt Avoid climbing ladders Hold handrails on stairs Never text while walking or driving
T is for Toxins Research shows marijuana users have low blood flow to the brain, and after a night of heavy drinking people have poorer attention, coordination, memory, and impaired reaction time when operating a moving vehicle.	Smoking Recreational/illicit drugs Alcohol Mold Pesticides Toxic products	Avoid toxic exposure and support the 4 organs of detoxification: <ul><li>*Kidneys – drink more water*</li><li>*Gut – eat more fiber and choose organic foods*</li><li>*Liver – quit smoking and doing drugs, limit alcohol, eat brassicas (cabbage, broccoli, cauliflower, and Brussels sprouts)*</li><li>*Skin – sweat with exercise and take saunas*</li></ul> Get tested for mold exposure Download the 'Think Dirty' app to scan your personal products to know if they're toxic
M is for Mind-Storms 1 in 5 US adults experiences mental health issues. (NAMI)	Depression Anxiety disorders Posttraumatic stress disorder Chronic stress ADD/ADHD	Adopt brain healthy habits ANT Therapy Exercise Increase omega-3 fatty acids
I is for Immunity/Infections COVID-19 survivors are at risk for depression and anxiety.	Low vitamin D level Lyme disease COVID-19 Autoimmune disorders, such as multiple sclerosis	Boost vitamin D intake and eat onions, mushrooms, and garlic Work with an integrative or functional medicine doctor who can properly diagnose and treat you
N is for Neurohormone Issues Neurohormones play a critical role in health and well-being.	Abnormal thyroid, DHEA, testosterone, estrogen, and progesterone in females	Test and optimize your hormones

Factors	Risks	Happy Brain Habits
D is for Diabesity Amen Clinics has published 3 studies showing that as weight goes up the size and function of the brain goes down.	Diabetes (high fasting blood sugar) Being overweight or obese (high BMI)	Follow the 13 Rules for Happy Eating (see Day 5).
Sleep Problems 60 million Americans have sleep-related issues.	Insomnia Sleep apnea	Target 7-8 hours Get an evaluation for sleep apnea if you snore Practice good sleep hygiene

Today's exercise: *Discover your BRIGHT MINDS risk factors by taking the Memory Rescue Assessment at https://memoryrescue.com/assessment.*

"Brain health is the missing link to happiness." — Daniel G. Amen, MD

DAY 4. WHY NUTRACEUTICALS?
(Relates to Secret 3)

To stay on track in your happiness journey, you need to give your brain a daily dose of nutrients. Considering most of us don't get adequate amounts of these important vitamins and minerals from the foods we eat, it's important to take nutritional supplements, or nutraceuticals. Why nutraceuticals? SPECT scans show that many psychiatric medications—such as benzodiazepines for anxiety, sleeping medications, and opiates for pain—have toxic effects on brain function. Science-based natural supplements can be an effective alternative without the toxic effects.

The basics every Brain Type needs to be happy include:

- **Multivitamin/Minerals:** In a 2020 review of the science on broad-spectrum nutritional supplements for the treatment of certain mental health issues, 16 of 23 studies showed positive effects for symptoms of depression, anxiety, or stress.

- **Omega-3 fatty acids:** When it comes to overall health and well-being, omega-3 fatty acids are essential. Insufficient levels of two of the most important omega-3s—eicosapentaenoic acid (EPA) and docosahexaenoic acid (DHA)—have also been linked to depression, bipolar disorder, suicidal behavior, ADHD, cognitive impairment, dementia, obesity, heart disease, and inflammation. An estimated 95% of Americans do not get enough dietary omega-3 fatty acids.

- **Probiotics:** If you're not happy, it may be related to your gut, which is often referred to as the "second brain." Considering the nearly 100 million neurons in the GI tract and the direct communication it has with the brain, the health of your gut is tightly linked to brain health and mental wellness.

- **Vitamin D:** This vitamin is critical for building bones and boosting the immune system, but it also is essential for a healthy brain, mood, and memory. Over 93% of Americans are low in vitamin D. Check your level and optimize it if necessary.

In addition, it's critical to take supplements to optimize your brain function based on your Brain Type. Taking supplements targeted to your Brain Type is the key because nutraceuticals that work for one Brain Type may not be effective for another type. See the chart below for supplements recommended for the 5 primary Brain Types.

Brain Type	Reccommended Supplements	BrainMD Solutions
Basics for All Types	Multivitamin/Minerals Omega-3 fatty acids Probiotics Vitamin D	Brain and Body Power Omega-3 Power ProBrainBiotics Vitamin D3
1. Balanced	Basic	Basic
2. Spontaneous	Basics + rhodiola, ginseng, green tea extract, ashwagandha, and L-tyrosine	Basics + Focus and Energy
3. Persistent	Basics + boost serotonin with 5HTP and B6	Basics + Serotonin Mood Support
4. Sensitive	Basics + saffron, curcumins, and zinc	Basics + Happy Saffron Plus or SAMe + Betaine TMG
5. Cautious	Basics + boost GABA to calm stress	Basics + GABA Calming Support

Today's exercise: *Nourish your brain with supplements for your Brain Type. You can order directly from BrainMD at* brainmd.com *or from your favorite high-quality supplement retailer.*

"If you're too happy, you must've had saffron." — Persian folklore

DAY 5. HAPPY FOODS
(Relates to Secret 4)

Today is a very important one in your journey, as you'll discover the 13 Rules for Happy Eating.

1. Choose foods that make you happy now *and* later.

2. Make your calories count toward happiness, not depression.

3. Hydrate to be happier.

4. Power up feel-good neurochemicals with high-quality protein.

5. Keep your brain happy with healthy fats. Low-fat diets are associated with risk of depression.

6. Opt for mood-boosting smart carbs (high in fiber, low in sugar).

7. Find happiness in your spice cabinet. Saffron boosts happiness. Cinnamon has been shown to be a natural aphrodisiac and helps with focus. Turmeric helps decrease inflammation.

8. Say yes to sexy foods—anything with cinnamon.

9. Eat clean to keep your body happy. Avoid processed foods with additives and sugary foods.

10. Fight depression and other happiness-draining issues with a month-long elimination diet. Eliminate gluten, dairy, corn, soy, artificial dyes, and sweeteners.

11. Disrupt hedonic adaptation with intermittent fasting.

12. Develop a happier mindset about your relationship with food. Only choose foods that love you back.

13. Eat for your Brain Type. (See chart below.)

Brain Type	How To Eat
1. Balanced	Balanced diet: high-quality proteins, complex carbohydrates (low-glycemic, high-fiber)
2. Spontaneous	Higher protein, lower simple carb diet
3. Persistent	Higher complex carbohydrate, lower protein diet
4. Sensitive	Balanced diet: high-quality proteins, complex carbohydrates (low-glycemic, high-fiber)
5. Cautious	Balanced diet: high-quality proteins, complex carbohydrates (low-glycemic, high-fiber)

Today's exercise: Choose 20 foods you love that love you back from the following list of Happy Foods. Circle your favorite foods or highlight them with a marker.

HAPPY FOODS AND BEVERAGES

Beverages

1. Beet juice (to increase blood flow)

2. Cherry juice (to help sleep)

3. Coconut water

4. Herbal Tea

5. Lightly flavored waters, such as Hint

6. Spa water – sparkling water with berries, a sprig of mint, or a slice of lemon, orange, peach, or melon

7. Sparkling water (add a splash of chocolate or orange stevia [brand: Sweet Leaf] for a refreshing, calorie- and toxin-free "soda")

8. Unsweetened almond milk (for amazing taste, add a few drops of flavored stevia)

9. Vegetable juice or green drinks (without added fruit juice)

10. Water

11. Water with cayenne pepper to boost metabolism

Nuts, Seeds, Nut and Seed Butter, and Meal

1. Almonds, raw
2. Almond flour
3. Almond butter
4. Brazil nuts
5. Cacao, raw
6. Cashews
7. Cashew butter
8. Chia seeds
9. Coconut
10. Flax seeds
11. Flax meal
12. Hemp seeds
13. Pistachios
14. Pumpkin Seeds
15. Sesame Seeds
16. Walnuts
17. Quinoa

Legumes (small amounts, all high in fiber and protein, help balance blood sugar)

1. Black Beans
2. Chickpeas
3. Green peas
4. Hummus
5. Kidney beans
6. Lentils
7. Navy beans
8. Pinto beans

Fruits (choose low-glycemic, high-fiber varieties)

1. Acai berries
2. Apples
3. Apricots
4. Avocados
5. Blackberries
6. Blueberries
7. Cantaloupe
8. Cherries
9. Cranberries
10. Figs
11. Goldenberries
12. Goji berries
13. Grapefruit
14. Grapes (red and green)
15. Honeydew melon
16. Kiwi
17. Kumquat
18. Lemons
19. Lychee
20. Mangosteen
21. Nectarines
22. Olives
23. Oranges
24. Passion fruit
25. Peaches
26. Pears
27. Plums
28. Pomegranates
29. Pumpkin
30. Raspberries
31. Strawberries
32. Tangerines
33. Tomatoes

Vegetables

1. Artichokes
2. Arugula
3. Asparagus
4. Beets and beet greens
5. Bell peppers
6. Broccoli
7. Brussels sprouts
8. Butter lettuce
9. Butternut squash
10. Cabbage
11. Carrots
12. Cauliflower
13. Celery
14. Celery root
15. Chicory
16. Chlorella
17. Collard greens
18. Cucumber
19. Garlic
20. Green beans
21. Horseradish
22. Jicama
23. Kale
24. Leeks
25. Maca root
26. Mustard greens
27. Okra
28. Onions
29. Parsley
30. Parsnips
31. Red or green leaf lettuce
32. Romaine lettuce
33. Scallions
34. Seaweed
35. Spinach
36. Spirulina
37. Summer squash
38. Sweet potatoes
39. Swiss chard
40. Turnips
41. Watercress
42. Wheatgrass juice
43. Zucchini

Prebiotic Foods

1. Artichokes
2. Asparagus
3. Beans
4. Cabbage
5. Chia Seeds
6. Dandelion greens
7. Dandelion greens
8. Leeks
9. Onions
10. Psyllium
11. Raw garlic
12. Root vegetables (including sweet potatoes, yams, squash, jicama, beets, carrots, and turnips)

Probiotic Foods

1. Brined vegetables (not vinegar)
2. Chlorella
3. Kefir
4. Kimchi
5. Kombucha tea
6. Miso Soup
7. Pickles
8. Sauerkraut (fresh)
9. Spirulina

Mushrooms

1. Black truffles
2. Chaga
3. Chanterelle
4. Maitake
5. Oyster
6. Porcini
7. Reishi
8. Shitake
9. Shimeji
10. White button

Oils

1. Avocado oil
2. Coconut oil (stable at high temperatures)
3. Macadamia nut oil
4. Olive oil (stable only at room temperature)

Eggs/Meat/Poultry/Fish

1. Arctic char
2. Chicken or turkey
3. Eggs
4. King Crab
5. Lamb (high in omega 3s)
6. Rainbow Trout
7. Salmon, wild caught
8. Sardines, wild caught
9. Scallops
10. Shrimp

Brain Healthy Herbs and Spices

1. Basil
2. Black pepper
3. Cayenne pepper
4. Cinnamon
5. Cloves
6. Curcumin
7. Garlic
8. Ginger
9. Marjoram
10. Mint
11. Nutmeg
12. Oregano
13. Parsley
14. Peppermint
15. Rosemary
16. Saffron
17. Sage
18. Thyme
19. Turmeric

Special Category

1. Shiratake noodles (the root of a wild yam plant—brand name Miracle Noodles—to replace pasta noodles)

"Eating crappy food isn't a reward—it's a punishment." — *Comedian, Drew Carey*

DAY 6. MASTER YOUR MIND
(Relates to Secret 5)

You've already reached Day 6 of your journey to getting happier! By now, you should be feeling the beneficial effects that come from enhancing your brain health and understanding your Brain Type. Despite your progress, you may still have some doubts about your ability to be a happy person. Today's lesson will help you combat those negative thoughts.

At Amen Clinics, we have found that people who struggle with unhappiness, anxiety, depression, and stress tend to have a very high negativity bias. This means having a tendency to see what's wrong in a situation, which contributes to negativity. Today, you're going to learn how to flip that to bring more positivity into your life.

Positivity bias training is a strategy that can help you train your brain to look for what's right, rather than what's wrong. Research shows that positivity bias training strategies help you overcome negative feelings and boost happiness. Today, you're going to learn one of the most ridiculously simple positivity bias strategies that can put you in a more positive mindset from the time you wake up.

All you have to do is to start your day by saying the following phrase:

"Today is going to be a great day."

I do this every morning. How does it work? It helps direct the unconscious mind to look for why it will be a great day and prevents it from seeking out what will go wrong.

As you already learned on Day 1, Question 5 is "What went well today?" Each night when you go to bed, you need to ask yourself this question. This is another positivity bias training exercise that lets you focus on the positives in your day and helps prepare your brain for more restful sleep and happier dreams.

Since you have already seen this question in you daily journal, use today to focus on starting a morning ritual that will spark a positive mindset.

Today's exercise: Start each day by saying, "Today is going to be a great day."

"Where you bring your attention determines how you feel." — Daniel G. Amen, MD

DAY 7. WHY I COLLECT PENGUINS
(Relates to Secret 6)

Up until now, your journey has mainly been focusing on yourself. Today, you're going to discover that how you view others also contributes to your happiness (or unhappiness). This is where Secret 6 comes in: Notice what you like about others more than what you don't. There's scientific proof that this works. Check out these statistics:

- Married couples who give each other 5 times more positive comments than negative ones are **_significantly less likely to get divorced._**

- Workers who exchange 5 times more positive comments than negative ones are **_significantly more likely to be high performing._**

Curious how I learned this secret? Here's my story:

About 37 years ago, I was a child psychiatry fellow, learning to be a child psychiatrist. My 7-year-old son was argumentative and oppositional, and it was very frustrating. To work on bonding with him, I took him to a place called Sea Life Park. We went to the penguin show because he wanted to see Fat Freddy, a penguin who did all sorts of amazing tricks.

During the show, the trainer asked Freddy to go get something, and Freddy went and got it and brought it right back. The world stopped for me in that moment because I knew if I asked my son to get something for me, he'd want to have a discussion for 20 minutes and then he wouldn't want to do it. And I knew my son was smarter than the penguin.

So, I went up to the trainer afterwards and asked how she got Freddy to do all these really cool things, and she said, "Unlike parents, whenever Freddy does anything the way I want him to do, I notice him. I give him a hug and I give him a fish."

The light went on in my head, and it became crystal clear to me that I was noticing what was wrong and what my son didn't do way more than when he did what was right. He behaved poorly to get my attention.

When I started noticing what my son did right, our relationship changed dramatically for the better, and we both were much happier. That's when I started collecting penguins, which represents the Social Circle (one of the 4 Circles of Happiness).

Today's exercise: *Write down 3 things you notice that you like about someone in your life.*

1. ____

2. ____

3. ____

"It is a wise thing to be polite; consequently, it is a stupid thing to be rude. To make enemies by unnecessary and willful incivility, is just as insane as to set your house on fire."
— *Arthur Schopenhauer*

DAY 8. CHOOSE YOUR VALUES
(Relates to Secret 7)

Congrats on starting week 2 of your happiness journey! I've found that many people are filled with enthusiasm in the first few days of their journey, but then it begins to wane. To help you stay motivated for the full 30 days and beyond, you need to know why you care. Knowing your core values is a key piece that helps you stay focused on what is important to you.

Step 1. Choose your important personal characteristics.
Circle 1-2 of the following traits in each of the four columns or feel free to add your own.

Biological	Psychological	Social	Spiritual
Athleticism	Authenticity	Caring	Acceptance
Beauty	Confidence	Connection	Appreciation
Brain Health	Courage	Dependability	Awareness (Awe)
Energy	Creativity	Empathy	Compassion
Focus	Flexibility	Encouragement	Generosity
Fitness	Forthrightness	Family	Gratitude
Longevity	Fun	Friendships	Growth
Love - Brain/Body	Happiness/Joy	Independence	Humility
Mental clarity	Hard work	Kindness	Inspiration
Physical health	Individuality	Love of others	Love/relationship w/God
Safety	Love-self	Loyalty	Morality
Strength	Open-minded	Outcome driven/service	Patience
Vitality	Positivity	Passion	Prayerful
	Resilience	Significance	Purposeful
	Responsibility	Success	Religious community
	Science-based	Tradition	Surrender
	Security		Transcendence
	Self-control		Wonder

Step 2. Look into your heroes.

Think of 6-8 heroes (past and present) you admire most in life and write down the values you think represent their lives. Heroes can be people you know personally, public figures, or even entities (such as a fire department or sports team)—anyone who has inspired you. Write them down in the chart below:

Hero	Values They Represent

Step 3: Review your values.

Observe yourself and learn over time what values you want and how they impact your life. Write them down and post them where you can see them often. Make it a habit to review your values from time to time to see if they still resonate with you or if you should update them.

Today's exercise: *Identify your core values by using the 3 steps described above.*

"You must know your 'why' in order to do the 'what' of getting and staying healthy." —Tana Amen, BSN, RN

DAY 9. KNOW YOUR PURPOSE
(Relates to Secret 7)

Today's lesson builds on what you learned yesterday. Knowing what your purpose is and what gives your life meaning is critically important to feeling content, satisfied, and fulfilled in life. Research shows that people who are more purposeful have greater happiness and less depression. Plus, they have more satisfaction, better mental health, personal growth, self-acceptance, longevity—and they sleep better!

How can you find your true purpose in life? You simply need to know where to look. To help you zero in on what gives your life meaning, write down your answers to the following 6 questions.

1. Look inward. *What do you love to do? Examples include writing, cooking, design, parenting, creating, speaking, teaching, and so on. What do you feel qualified to teach others about?*

____

____

2. Look outward. *Who do you do it for? How does your work connect you to others?*

____

____

3. Look back. *Who do you do it for? How does your work connect you to others?*

____

____

4. Look beyond yourself. *What do others want or need from you?*

____

____

5. Look for transformation. *How do others change as a result of what you do?*

---

6. Look to the end. *Psychiatrist Elisabeth Kubler-Ross, author of On Death and Dying, said, "It is the denial of death that is partially responsible for people living empty, purposeless lives; for when you live as if you'll live forever, it becomes too easy to postpone the things you know that you must do." Ask yourself, "Does this worry, problem or moment have eternal value? When I die, how do I want to be remembered?"*

Notice that only 2 of the 6 questions are about you; 4 of them are about others. Happiness is often found in helping others.

Today's exercise: *Discover your purpose by answering the 6 questions.*

> *"If you want happiness for an hour, take a nap.*
> *If you want happiness for a day, go fishing.*
> *If you want happiness for a year, inherit a fortune.*
> *If you want happiness for a lifetime, help somebody."*
> — *A wise Chinese saying*

DAY 10. ONE PAGE MIRACLE
(Relates to Secret 7)

Now that you know your core values and your purpose, it's time to look ahead to your goals in life. Today's strategy centers on a life-changing exercise called the One Page Miracle (OPM) that helps you identify your goals. Basically, you ask yourself what you want (not what you don't want) in the 4 Circles of your life—biological, psychological, social, and spiritual. When you tell your brain what you want, your brain will help you make it happen. The OPM will help guide your thoughts, words, and behaviors. It's a powerful tool for all Brain Types and can be especially beneficial for the Spontaneous Brain Type.

Here's how it looks when I answered these questions about my goals.

Biological Goals: What do I want for my brain and body?
Dr. Amen's example: I want to be mentally sharp and physically strong for as long as possible. It is the foundation of my happiness, success, and independence.

Psychological Goals: What do I want for my mind?
Dr. Amen's example: I want to be happy, authentic, and able to manage my mind with positivity, while having enough anxiety to keep me on track.

Social Goals: What do I want for my relationships, work, school, and money?
Dr. Amen's example on relationship: I want a kind, caring, loving, supportive, passionate relationship with my spouse. If I have any rude thoughts in my head about my spouse or our relationship, I don't say them because they don't fit with what I want for my relationship.

Spiritual Goals: What do I want spiritually?
Dr. Amen's example: Be attentive to God's will in my life through daily prayer, do my part to keep the planet healthy, honor my ancestors, and nurture my grandchildren who are our future.

Today's exercise: *Fill out the OPM form with your core values, purpose, and goals. Then place it where you can see it every day, and routinely ask yourself if your behavior fits the goals you have for your life.*

"If we have our why of life we shall get along with almost any how."
— *Frederick Nietzsche*

One Page Miracle
Does It Fit?

Core Values

Biological: _______________
____

Psychological: _______________
____

Social: _______________
____

Spiritual: _______________
____

Purpose

____
____
____
____
____
____

Overall

Biological Goals
Brain and Body

____
____
____

3 Brain Health Strategies
Brain Envy – test on regular basis
Avoid Bad – BRIGHT MINDS Risks
Do Good – BRIGHT MINDS Strategies

BRIGHT MINDS
Blood flow – exercise (walk like you are late for 10,000 steps a day)
Retirement/Aging – new learning
Inflammation – eliminate processed foods, floss, omega-3s and probiotics daily
Genetics – Know and prevent vulnerabilities
Head trauma – Protect my head
Toxins – avoid and support 4 organs of detoxification

Mental Health (see Psychological goals)
Immunity/Infections – optimize gut, Vitamin D level
Neurohormones – test and optimize regularly
Diabesity – Healthy weight and blood sugar
Sleep – 7-8 hours a night

Psychological Goals
Mind

____
____
____

Eliminate ANTs w/5 Questions
Write down the negative belief
Ask:
Is it true?
Is it absolutely true?
How do I feel with the thought?
How do I feel without the thought?
Is the opposite of the thought true or even truer than the original thought?

Social Goals
Relationships, Work, Money

Relationships

Partner_______________
____
Family _______________
____
Friends _______________
____

RELATING
Responsibility
Empathy
Listening
Assertiveness
Time
Inquire
Notice what you like
Grace/forgiveness

Work/School
____
____
____

Money
____
____
____

Spiritual Goals
Meaning and Purpose

God: _______________
____
____

Planet _______________
____
____

Connection to Past Generations _______________
____
____

Connection to Future Generations _______________
____
____

DAY 11. TAME YOUR DRAGONS
(Relates to Secret 5)

You may be surprised to realize that one of the keys to getting happier is knowing what makes you *unhappy*. On your happiness journey, you may be faced with unexpected setbacks that threaten your progress and make you feel down. These can be related to what I call the Dragons of the Past—the big emotional issues we have that are always breathing fire on our limbic (emotional) brain. When they are triggered by life events, these dragons can roar to life and stomp on your happiness.

I've identified 13 Dragons from the Past that contribute to unhappiness:

1. Abandoned, Invisible, or Insignificant Dragons—feel alone, unseen, or unimportant

2. Inferior or Flawed Dragons—feel inferior to others

3. Anxious Dragons—feel fearful and overwhelmed

4. Wounded Dragons—bruised by past trauma

5. Should and Shaming Dragons—racked with guilt

6. Special, Spoiled, or Entitled Dragons—feel more special than others

7. Responsible Dragons—need to take care of others

8. Angry Dragons—harbor hurts and rage

9. Judgmental Dragons—hold harsh or critical opinions of others due to past injustices

10. Death Dragons—fear the future and lack of a meaningful life

11. Grief and Loss Dragons—feel loss and fear of loss

12. Hopeless or Helpless Dragons—have pervasive sense of despair and discouragement

13. Ancestral Dragons—affected by issues from past generations

Today's exercise: *Take the Know Your Dragons Quiz at knowyourdragons.com to identify which dragons you have that are making you unhappy. Circle your dragons above.*

"People who deny the existence of dragons are often eaten by dragons. From within."
— Ursula K. Le Guin, The Wave in the Mind

DAY 12. WHY I COLLECT SEAHORSES
(Relates to Secret 2)

What do seahorses have to do with happiness? Let me explain.

I've collected seahorses ever since I wrote Memory Rescue in 2017. In my view, seahorses represent the Biological Circle (one of the 4 Circles of Happiness). Specifically, I collect them to honor a part of the brain called the hippocampus—the Greek translation is seahorse because of its shape. The hippocampus is a part of your limbic or emotional brain. It's involved in mood, memory, learning, and spatial awareness.

Underneath your temples and behind your eyes, the hippocampi (plural of hippocampus) are located on the inside of your left and right temporal lobes. They're so important, because every day—under the right circumstances—they make stem cells that create new brain cells (think baby seahorses) that become a part of the hippocampi.

New research suggests we can produce up to 700 new cells a day if we put them in a nourishing environment, meaning:

- **good nutrition**
- **omega-3 fatty acids**
- **oxygen**
- **blood flow**
- **stimulation**

If you nourish your brain and body, the hippocampi (seahorses) can grow stronger, but if your behavior hurts your biology, they will shrink.

***Today's exercise:** Circle 3 strategies out of the following 110 BRIGHT MINDS Ways to Grow Your Hippocampus to start today.*

<u>B</u>LOOD FLOW
1. Keep blood pressure optimized
2. Drink water—blood is mostly water
3. Limit caffeine and nicotine
4. Take up a racquet sport
5. Small piece of sugar-free dark chocolate
6. Ginkgo biloba, vinpocetine
7. Spice up your food: add cayenne pepper

8. Arginine rich foods, including beets
9. Magnesium rich foods, e.g. pumpkin seeds
10. Drink green tea

RETIREMENT/AGING

1. Limit charred meats
2. Get ferritin checked
3. Donate blood
4. Daily 12-16 hour fast
5. Cloves as a potent antioxidant
6. Acetyl-l-carnitine (ALCAR), huperzine A
7. Acetylcholine rich foods, such as shrimp
8. Stay connected, volunteer
9. Music training
10. Learn something new everyday

INFLAMMATION

1. Floss daily and care for your gums
2. Test CRP (c-reactive protein), Omega-3 Index; aim > 8%
3. Eliminate trans fats
4. Limit omega-6 rich foods (corn, soy, and processed foods)
5. Increase omega-3 rich foods (fish, Avocados, and walnuts)
6. Omega-3 supplements
7. Vitamins B6, B12 and folate
8. Fix leaky gut
9. Prebiotic foods
10. Probiotic foods and/or supplements

GENETICS

1. If you have genetic risk, be serious about brain health as soon as possible
2. Test your Apo E gene type
3. If you have Apo E4 gene avoid contact sports or other head trauma risks
4. Early screening with SPECT
5. Limit high-glycemic, saturated fat foods (pizza), processed cheeses,
and microwave popcorn
6. Curcumin - decrease amyloid plaques
7. Organic blueberries – clear amyloid plaques
8. Cook with sage-decrease amyloid plaques
9. Ginseng
10. CoQ 10

HEAD TRAUMA

1. Wear a seatbelt
2. Be thoughtful about actions
3. Wear a helmet when skiing, biking, etc.
4. Avoid going up on any roof unless it's safe
5. Slow down
6. Do not text and walk or drive
7. Hold the handrail when going downstairs
8. If you've had head trauma check your hormones
9. Peppermint herbs to help with healing
10. Hyperbaric oxygen therapy (HBOT)

TOXINS

1. Decrease exposure to pesticides, buy organic
2. Avoid fumes when pumping gas
3. Quit smoking, avoid secondhand smoke
4. Support kidneys: drink more water
5. Support liver: limit alcohol, increase NAC and brassicas (cabbage, cauliflower and Brussels sprouts)
6. Support gut health -eat more fiber
7. Support skin - sweat with exercise and saunas
8. Avoid handling cash register receipts (BPAs)
9. Don't drink or eat out of plastic containers
10. Use Think Dirty app to scan personal products to eliminate toxins

MENTAL HEALTH

1. Start every day with "Today is going to be a great day."
2. Write down 3 things you're grateful for daily
3. Worriers consider Serotonin Mood Support
4. Trouble with focus, consider higher protein, lower carbohydrate diet
and Focus and Energy (Is this referring to a Brain MD product, maybe we can link it)
5. Eat up to eight fruits and vegetables a day (linear correlation with happiness)
6. Meditation, e.g., "Loving Kindness Meditation"
7. Take a walk in nature link i
8. Saffron helps mood and memory
9. If natural interventions are ineffective, work with a local therapist or psychiatrist
10. Kill the ANTs (automatic negative thoughts)

IMMUNITY/INFECTION ISSUES

1. If struggling with memory issues, consider being tested for exposure to infections
2. Elimination diet for a month to see if food allergies may be damaging immune system
3. Avoid hiking where deer ticks and black-legged ticks live
4. Know and optimize vitamin D level

5. Add extra vitamin C
6. Supplement with aged garlic
7. Add onions
8. Add Shiitake mushrooms
9. Decrease alcohol -- Why do nurses swab alcohol on your skin before giving you a shot? To decrease the bacteria. Drinking excessive alcohol can upset the gut microbiome, which is critical to immunity.
10. Watch a comedy to boost immunity

<u>N</u>EUROHORMONE DEFICIENCIES
1. Test your hormones on a regular basis
2. Avoid hormone disruptors, such as BPAs, phthalates, parabens, and pesticides
3. Avoid animal proteins raised with hormones or antibiotics
4. Add fiber to decrease unhealthy estrogens
5. Lift weights to boost testosterone
6. Limit sugar which disrupts hormones
7. Zinc to help boost testosterone
8. Cortisol reducing supplements, such as ashwagandha (also supports thyroid)
9. For women, optimize estrogen
10. Hormone replacement when needed

<u>D</u>IABESITY
1. Know your BMI and check it monthly
2. Measure your Waist-to-Height Ratio
3. Don't drink your calories
4. Start the Memory Rescue Diet
5. Have protein and fat at each meal to stabilize blood sugar and cravings
6. Lose weight slowly if you are overweight (develop lifelong habits)
7. Chromium picolinate
8. Alpha lipoic acid
9. Cinnamon spice
10. Nutmeg spice

<u>S</u>LEEP ISSUES
1. If you snore, get assessed for sleep apnea
2. Eliminate caffeine during the day
3. Put blue light blockers on your gadgets
4. Cool your home a bit before bedtime
5. Darken your room
6. Turn off gadgets at night
7. Maintain a regular sleep schedule
8. Melatonin and magnesium
9. Listen to a hypnosis sleep audio
10. 5HTP if you are a worrier

Yesterday, I told you why I collect seahorses. Today, I want to tell you about my anteater collection and how an anteater can help you conquer negativity. I started collecting anteaters about 30 years ago. On a very trying day after seeing 4 suicidal patients, 2 teen runaways, and 2 couples who hated each other, I came home to an ant infestation. As I was cleaning them up, I had the epiphany that my patients' minds were infested with ANTs (automatic negative thoughts). I went to a puppet store and found an anteater puppet, and my anteater collection was born. The anteaters are representative of the Psychological Circle (one of the 4 Circles of Happiness) and serve as a reminder that you don't have to believe every stupid thought you have.

Learning how to challenge your ANTs and gain control of your thinking is a foundational principle for happiness.

Here are 9 types of ANT species you need to know:

- **All or Nothing:** Thinking things are all good or all bad
- **Less Than:** Where you compare and see yourself as less than others
- **Just the Bad:** Seeing only the bad in a situation
- **Guilt Beating:** Thinking in words like should, must, ought, or have to
- **Labeling:** Attaching a negative label to yourself or someone else
- **Fortune Telling:** Predicting the worst possible outcome
- **Mind Reading:** Believing you know what others are thinking
- **If Only and I'll Be Happy When:** Where you argue with the past and long for the future
- **Blaming:** Blaming someone or something else for your problems

Learn to Kill the ANTs

Whenever you feel mad, sad, nervous, or out of control, write down what you're thinking and identify the ANT species. Then ask yourself these 5 questions that I learned from Byron Katie:

1. Is it true?
2. Is it absolutely true with 100% certainty?

3. How do I feel when I believe this thought?
4. How would I feel if I couldn't think this thought?
5. Turn the thought around to its exact opposite, and then ask yourself if the opposite of the thought is true or even truer than the original thought.

Answering these 5 questions is about accurate and honest thinking and telling yourself the truth without the negative noise. Look at the example below to see how it's done.

ANT KILLING EXAMPLES

Example #1: *During the pandemic, one of my patients called in a panic because she lost her job and said:*

"I'll never be able to work again."

ANT: *I'll never be able to work again.*

ANT Type(s): Fortune-Telling

1. Is it true? Yes.

2. Is it absolutely true with 100 percent certainty? No, I already have part-time work lined up.

3. How do I feel when I believe this thought? Trapped, victimized, helpless.

4. How would I feel if I couldn't have the thought? Massively relieved, happy, joyful, free, like my usual self.

5. Turn the thought around to its exact opposite: I can get work again.
Any evidence that that's true? I have valuable skills that will help me get a job.

Thought to meditate on: *I have valuable skills that will help me get a job.*

Today's exercise: *Learn to kill the ANTs using the 5 questions then challenge 100 of your worst thoughts. You don't have to kill all 100 ANTs today. Start by killing 3 ANTs today using the forms below and work through a few more of them each day for the remainder of this 30-day journey.*

*ANT #1*____

ANT Type (s):____

1. Is it true?
2. Is it 100% true?
3. How do you feel when you believe that thought?
4. Without the thought?
5. Opposite:

Meditation: ____

*ANT #2*____

ANT Type (s):____

1. Is it true?
2. Is it 100% true?
3. How do you feel when you believe that thought?
4. Without the thought?
5. Opposite:

Meditation: ____

*ANT #3*____

ANT Type (s):____

1. Is it true?
2. Is it 100% true?
3. How do you feel when you believe that thought?
4. Without the thought?
5. Opposite:

Meditation: ____

"Mental hygiene is as important as washing your hands"
— Daniel G. Amen, MD

DAY 14. WHY I COLLECT BUTTERFLIES
(Relates to Secret 7)

To me, butterflies represent the Spiritual Circle (one of the 4 Circles of Happiness). Not only are they beautiful and graceful, but they're also a symbol of transformation. I've had the privilege to witness many transformations at Amen Clinics. My best-selling book of all time is called *Change Your Brain, Change Your Life*. When I wrote it, I had come to realize that you are not stuck with the brain you have. You can transform it. You can make your brain better by doing the right things—and with a better brain, you're much happier. And that's why I started collecting butterflies.

One of the ways to help your transformation to being a happier person is to know why you want to become happier. Examples may include:

- **Yourself**
- **Your family**
- **Your work or business**
- **Your community**
- **Your church**

Photos or videos of the people, places, or things that are driving you to be happier can help. These are called anchor images. About 50% of your brain is visual, so your anchor images are visual cues that are powerful reminders of what motivates you. They can help you in your journey to be healthier and happier.

Today's exercise: *Pick 4-5 anchor images you can put on your phone or in your home to remind yourself every day what or who is motivating you to be happier.*

"Change your brain, change your life."
— *Daniel G. Amen, MD*

DAY 15. SLEEP YOUR WAY TO HAPPINESS
(Relates to Secret 2)

You've made it through 2 weeks of your happiness journey! Up until now, you've been focusing on using your days to actively ramp up your happiness levels. Today, you're going to switch to focusing on helping your brain get the rest it needs.

Sleep is so important to happiness but many of us aren't getting enough of it. About 60 million Americans have sleep-related problems, including chronic insomnia, sleep apnea, and taking sleeping pills (which train your brain to need them in order for you to feel normal).

How does sleep affect happiness?

* People who get less than 6 or 7 hours of sleep have lower overall blood flow to the brain—they have more **brain fog** and make **worse decisions**.
* The risk of developing **depression** is 5 times higher in people with insomnia.
* People with insomnia are 20 times more likely to develop **anxiety disorders.**
* When adults sleep less than 8 hours, 40% report feeling **overwhelmed.**
* Poor sleep also **takes a toll** on relationships, parenting, work, performance, and cognitive performance.
* Sleep apnea may increase the risk of **Alzheimer's disease.**

Look at the following sleep dos and don'ts to learn how you can improve your sleep

Sleep Do's and Dont's

20 Sleep Enhancers

1. Keep your bedroom cool.

2. Make your bedroom completely dark or wear an eye mask.

3. Make the room noise free or wear ear plugs.

4. Turn off phones and other gadgets by the bed, or at least turn off the sound.

5. Try to fix emotional problems before going to sleep with a positive text, email, or intention to deal with the issues tomorrow.

6. Maintain a regular sleep schedule—going to bed at the same time each night and waking up at the same time each day, including on weekends.

7. Get up the same day regardless of sleep duration the previous night.

8. Create a soothing nighttime routine that encourages sleep. A warm bath, meditation, or massage can help you relax.

9. Some people like to read themselves to sleep. If you are reading, make sure it isn't an action-packed thriller or a horror story—they aren't likely to help you drift off to sleep.

10. Sound therapy can induce a very peaceful mood and lull you to sleep. Consider soothing nature sounds, wind chimes, a fan, or soft music. You can find sleep enhancing music by Grammy award winning producer Barry Goldstein on BrainFitLife.

11. Drink a mixture of warm unsweetened almond milk, a teaspoon of vanilla (the real stuff, not imitation), and a few drops of stevia. This may increase serotonin in your brain and help you sleep.

12. Take a warm bath or shower before bed.

13. Wear socks to bed. Researchers have found that warm hands and feet were the best predictor of rapid sleep onset.

14. If you wake up in the middle of the night, refrain from looking at the clock. Checking the time can make you feel anxious, which aggravates the problem.

15. Use the bed and bedroom only for sleep or sexual activity. Sexual activity releases many natural hormones, releases muscle tension, and boosts a sense of well-being. Adults with healthy sex lives tend to sleep better. When you are unable to fall asleep or return to sleep easily, get up and go to another room.

16. Talk to your doctor if you're taking any medications that can disrupt sleep, such as asthma medications, antihistamines, cough medicines, anticonvulsants, or stimulants prescribed for ADD/ADHD.

17. When you go to bed, ask yourself, "What went well today?" This will help set you up for more pleasant dreams and better sleep.

18. Hypnosis or meditation can help. We have audio downloads on BrainMD.com that could be helpful.

19. Use the scent of lavender to enhance sleep. It has been shown to decrease anxiety, improve mood, and help with relaxation.

20. Natural supplements, such as BrainMD's Put Me to Sleep or Restful Sleep may be helpful.

20 Sleep Stealers

1. Don't eat for at least 2-3 hours before going to bed.

2. Don't exercise within 4 hours of the time you hit the sack. Vigorous exercise late in the evening may energize you and keep you awake.

3. Don't keep your room warm.

4.   Don't have lights on in the bedroom.

5.   Don't sleep in a noisy environment.

6.   Don't keep tech gadgets by the bed.

7.   Don't go to bed worried or angry.

8.   If you are having trouble sleeping, don't take naps! This is one of the biggest mistakes you can make if you have insomnia. Taking naps when you feel sleepy during the day compounds the nighttime sleep cycle disruption.

9.   Avoid caffeine. Too much caffeine from coffee, tea, chocolate, or some herbal preparations, especially when consumed later in the day or at night, can disrupt sleep.

10.   Skip alcohol, nicotine, and marijuana. Although these compounds initially induce sleepiness for some people, they have the reverse effect as they wear off, which is why you may wake up several hours after you go to sleep.

11.   Don't ignore medical conditions, such as thyroid conditions. congestive heart failure, acid reflux, chronic pain conditions, or restless leg syndrome.

12.   Don't ignore snoring or sleep apnea.

13.   Don't ignore women's issues, such as pregnancy, PMS, menopause, or perimenopause that cause fluctuations in hormone levels that can disrupt the sleep cycle.

14.   Don't ignore men's issues, such as benign prostatic hypertrophy, which causes many trips to the bathroom at night and interrupts slumber.

15.   Don't ignore psychiatric conditions such as obsessive-compulsive disorder, depression, or anxiety that can impact sleep.

16.   Don't ignore the fact that Alzheimer's disease patients "sundown" or rev up at night and wander.

17.   Don't let shift work ruin your sleep. Develop a routine that promotes good sleep patterns regardless of your work schedule.

18.   Don't let stressful events steal your sleep.

19.   When traveling, don't let jet lag ruin your sleep if at all possible.

20.   f you have to resort to medication, stay away from the benzodiazepines and traditional sleep medications.

Today's exercise: *Go to bed 30 minutes earlier tonight.*

"If you want to improve your brain and feel better tomorrow, improve your sleep tonight." — Daniel G. Amen, MD

DAY 16. GIVE YOUR MIND A NAME
(Relates to Secret 5)

I hope your brain got a good night's rest last night! Today, we're going to take a deep dive inside your brain to investigate why so many of us have a constant stream of unhelpful thoughts bouncing around our brains. Where do these thoughts come from? They can come from your emotional chains, from the news, from what your parents said, and from your boss, siblings, and friends. Thoughts come from all sorts of places, but you don't have to attach to them. In fact, it's not the thoughts you have that make you suffer. It's the thoughts you attach to that make you suffer.

I learned a great exercise from a friend of mine, Steven C. Hayes, Ph.D., author of A Liberated Mind. It's called "Give Your Mind a Name." Basically, you give your internal voice a name that you don't call yourself. If your mind has a different name, then it's different from "you." And it works!

What would you call your mind?

I have a name for my mind: Hermie.

That was the name of my beloved pet racoon when I was a kid. Hermie was a troublemaker—just like my own mind. Even after all these years, at times Hermie still holds up signs like, "You're an idiot," "You're a failure," or "Wow, you could have done that better." When Hermie would get out of control, I would put her in her cage. Now, when Hermie causes trouble in my mind, I metaphorically put her in her cage for a while.

Decades of research show that talking to yourself inside of your head this way, which is known as "distanced self-talk," can foster psychological distance and lead to:
- **better emotional regulation**
- **greater self-control**
- **more wisdom**

Today's exercise: Give your mind a name and write it below.

____

"You are NOT your mind." — Daniel G. Amen, MD

DAY 17. INTERRUPT UNNECESSARY UNHAPPY MOMENTS *(Relates to Secret 5)*

Because your thoughts are so important to your happiness (or unhappiness), we're going to continue exploring them today. And you're going to learn how to stop random unhappy musings from ruining your day with a great exercise I learned from my friend Joseph McClendon III. When he was a teenager, a racially motivated attack by 3 white men left him injured and eventually homeless. After hitting rock bottom, he somehow transformed his mindset to become a doctor of neuropsychology, a bestselling author, and a spell-binding orator who often teaches at Tony Robbins' seminars.

Whenever you notice you're having repetitive, unhappy times or repetitive unhappy feelings, follow this simple—but powerful— 4-step process to get you back on track:

Step 1. Feel bad on purpose.
- Spend a few seconds feeling bad; go to that dark place.
- Let the bad feeling wash over you.
- Sounds sort of crazy, but if you know how to make yourself feel bad, you can also decide to interrupt it. That's empowering.

Step 2. Interrupt the pattern.
- Say "Stop!"
- Stand up, or if you're not able to, turn your head or wave your arms or hands.
- Take 3 deep breaths.
- By doing this, you create space where a momentary void will occur.

Step 3. Purposely focus on happy memories.
- Fill the void with a happy memory so you can feel good on purpose. Remember, where you bring your attention always determines how you feel.
- Write down 10-20 of your happiest life memories, so you can recall one of them while doing this exercise.
- After you stand up, focus on one of those nice memories with all of your senses until you can truly feel happy or joyful.

Step 4. Celebrate!
- Wire the good feeling in your nervous system by celebrating your ability to interrupt the unnecessary, unhappy moments.

***Today's exercise:** Think of 2-3 things that repeatedly bother you and do these 4 steps with each of them.*

"Interrupt unnecessary unhappy moments." — Joseph McClendon III

DAY 18. PLAY THE GLAD GAME
(Relates to Secrets 5 and 6)

Now that you're getting the hang of controlling your thoughts, it's time to tackle how to shift your mindset. An excellent example of how to do this comes from the movie, Pollyanna, which was one of my favorite Disney films growing up. In the film, the main character, Pollyanna, tells her friends that her departed father came up with something called the "Glad Game." It came about after Pollyanna received a pair of crutches in the mail instead of the doll she had requested for Christmas. It would be understandable for Pollyanna to be sad or upset about the mix-up. But her dad challenged her to think about what there was that she could be glad about instead. After thinking for a moment, Pollyanna said she was thankful that she didn't need the crutches. Pollyanna started playing the Glad Game on a regular basis. Her philosophy about finding something to be glad about in any situation is an excellent way to go through life.

No matter what situation or setback you find yourself in, ask yourself this question:

What is there to be glad about?

Even during a pandemic, you can find things to be glad about, such as:

- Feeling closer to children due to more time together
- Rediscovering the after-dinner walk
- Eating more home-cooked meals and less fast food
- Playing board games together or taking up new hobbies like woodworking or knitting
- Practicing a musical instrument that had been gathering dust for years
- Rediscovering reading
- Going to bed earlier
- Going on local hikes
- Less traffic on the highways
- Having time to re-evaluate values
- How about you? What things are you glad about? When it comes to being happy, it's a good idea to start training your mind to look for what's right, rather than what's wrong.

How about you? What things are you glad about? When it comes to being happy, it's a good idea to start training your mind to look for what's right, rather than what's wrong.

Today's exercise: Play the Glad Game. Find something to be glad about today even if you're having a tough day.

"Pollyanna: A person characterized by irrepressible optimism and a tendency to find good in everything." — Merriam-Webster Dictionary

DAY 19. LOVING KINDNESS MEDITATION
(Relates to Secrets 2,5,6 and 7)

Gaining control of your mind is a big step toward happiness. But actively directing your thoughts can be even more powerful. For example, practicing meditation has been scientifically shown to increase your level of happiness. Loving Kindness Meditation is a form of meditation that is intended to develop feelings of goodwill and warmth toward others. It has been found to increase positive emotions and decrease negative ones, decrease pain and migraine headaches, reduce symptoms of PTSD, increase gray matter in the emotional processing areas of the brain, and boost social connectedness.

Here's How to do Loving Kindness Meditation
Sit in a comfortable position and close your eyes. Take 2-3 deep breaths, taking twice as long to exhale. Let any worries or concerns drift away and feel your breath moving through the area around your heart. As you sit, quietly or silently repeat the following or similar phrases:
> *May I be safe and secure*
> *May I be healthy and strong*
> *May I be happy and purposeful*
> *May I be at peace*

Let the intentions expressed in these phrases sink in as you repeat them. Allow the feelings to grow deeper. After you repeat them 10-20 times, direct the phrases to someone you feel grateful for or someone who has helped you:
> *May you be safe and secure*
> *May you be healthy and strong*
> *May you be happy and purposeful*
> *May you be at peace*

Next, visualize someone you feel neutral about. Choose among people you neither like nor dislike and repeat the phrases. After that, visualize someone you don't like or with whom you are having a hard time. Finally, direct the phrases toward everyone universally:
> *May you be safe and secure*
> *May you be healthy and strong*
> *May you be happy and purposeful*
> *May you be at peace*

You can do this for up to 30 minutes; it's up to you.

Today's exercise: *Practice Loving Kindness Meditation today.*

"Learn to be calm and you will always be happy." — *Paramahansa Yogananda*

DAY 20. GRATITUDE DAY
(Relates to Secret 5)

Today's happiness lesson focuses on gratitude. Expressing gratitude evokes strong feelings of positivity not only in the person who receives the recognition but also in the person who expresses appreciation. A wealth of research suggests that a daily practice of gratitude can improve your emotions, health, relationships, personality, and career.

Gratitude can enhance:
- Happiness and well-being
- Mood and optimism
- Self-esteem
- Resilience and resistance to stress
- Vitality and energy
- Help with longevity—and so much more

Gratitude helps direct your attention to positive feelings and away from negative ones.

I once did a study with Noel Nelson, looking at the power of gratitude and appreciation. She was writing a book and she wanted me to scan her brain while she was focusing on what she was grateful for in her life. When she focused on what she loved about her life her scan looked very healthy. A couple of days later, I scanned her when she focused on what she was not grateful for—what made her anxious, sad, and afraid. When she was focused on negativity, it decreased blood flow in parts of her brain.

Where you bring your attention determines how you feel, and it also determines how your brain works. When you focus on what you're grateful for, your brain works better. When you focus on what makes you anxious, nervous, sad, or afraid, your brain doesn't work as well, which then makes it harder to manage the things that make you feel anxious, sad, fearful, and afraid.

Today's exercise: *In the spaces below, list 10 things you are grateful for.*

________________________________   ________________________________

________________________________   ________________________________

________________________________   ________________________________

________________________________   ________________________________

________________________________   ________________________________

"If you want to find happiness, find gratitude." — Behavioral scientist Steve Maraboli, author of Unapologetically You

DAY 21. APPRECIATION DAY
(Relates to Secret 6)

Yesterday, you discovered how gratitude can boost happiness. Today, you're going to see how appreciation can take gratitude to a new level. So often, we take people and time for granted. That's a shame because expressing and showing heartfelt appreciation for others is such an easy way to boost happiness. Appreciation is like gratitude squared because it builds bridges between people and evokes positive feelings in the person who expresses the appreciation and the person who is on the receiving end. It's a win-win of happiness!

Think about a time when someone told you they appreciated something about you. How did that make you feel? When was the last time you let someone know how much you appreciated them? What emotions did that elicit?

Small gestures of appreciation can go a long way and are so easy to do. For example:

- Tell your significant other how much you appreciate the way their smile warms your heart.
- Thank your child for making you laugh today.
- Let a close friend know how much your friendship means to you and how much you love them.

When you consistently think about what you appreciate in others, you're being grateful. When you express your appreciation to them, it elevates the experience and boosts your happiness.

Today's exercise: *Send an appreciation text to someone today using one of the 20 sample appreciation texts below.*

20 Appreciation Texts You Can Send

1. I love the way you make me smile every time I see you

2. I wish everybody could have a positive attitude like you do.

3. Thanks for making me laugh today.

4. You are such an amazing mentor and a big part of my success.

5. When I have big news to tell, you're the first person I want to share it with.

6. Whenever I feel down, I know you'll support me. That means so much to me.

7. Have I told you lately how much I love you?

8. You're so awesome, you must have a beautiful brain!

9. Somebody asked me today who my role models are. You are the first person I mentioned.

10. I feel like I'm a better person when I'm around you.

11. With you in my life, I feel like I can do anything!

12. Wanna know a secret? I couldn't get by in this world without you

13. You make me feel like 😁 😍

14. 1You're the best. I wish I could clone you.

15. Thank you for letting me feel like I can be my 100% authentic self—quirks and all—around you.

16. Did you know that every day I thank God for putting you in my life?

17. Merci! Gracias! Danke! Thank you for being the only person like you in the whole wide world!

18. You may think nobody notices all the helpful things you do. You're wrong! I notice them every day.

19. You have the best quality in a coworker: You help make my job easier. Thank you!

20. I will always treasure your friendship…no matter how many miles separate us.

*"When you appreciate the good, the good appreciates." — Tal Ben-Shahar, author of
Choose the Life You Want: The Mindful Way to Happiness*

DAY 22. MICRO-MOMENTS OF HAPPINESS *(Relates to Secret 5 and 6)*

So far on your happiness journey you've been getting the big ideas about happiness. But today, it's time to focus on the small stuff. Some people mistakenly believe that joy can only be found in major life-changing events (getting married or having a baby), accomplishments (getting a new job or launching a business), or milestones (a wedding anniversary or your child's college graduation). While these may have a positive impact, your happiness is largely derived from the little things in life. Making the effort to notice and acknowledge the small stuff can dramatically increase your feelings of contentment on an everyday basis.

I call these Micro-Moments of Happiness. Here are a few examples:

- Hearing a bird sing outside your window
- Feeling the warmth of the sun on your face when you step outside
- Petting your dog or cat
- Getting a hug from your child
- Hearing a favorite old song play on the radio

It's so important to notice and savor the Micro-Moments of Happiness you experience because when your brain is paying attention to them, they add up to more overall satisfaction and fulfillment with your life.

Getting into the habit of looking for and finding the teeny-tiny, itty-bitty Micro-Moments of Happiness throughout your day trains your brain to have a positivity bias. It helps you appreciate the abundance of joy in your life and elevates your level of happiness.

Today's exercise: Notice and record 10 Micro-Moments of Happiness in your day. Write them below or use the notes section of your phone to record them throughout your day. Read them at the end of the day to make sure you don't miss out on the little things that help you feel happy.

__________________________________   __________________________________

__________________________________   __________________________________

__________________________________   __________________________________

__________________________________   __________________________________

__________________________________   __________________________________

"The more micro-moments you cherish, the greater your sense of joy."
— Daniel G. Amen, MD

DAY 23. MOOD AND MUSIC
(Relates to Secret 2, 5, and 6)

The majority of the feel-good strategies you have been learning so far center on developing happiness from within. Starting today, I'm going to introduce you to some ways you can use external stimuli to boost your moods. One of the best ways to do this is with music. Listening to music affects your thoughts and feelings, and research has shown that it can soothe, inspire, improve your mood, and help you focus. Brain imaging studies show that music also releases important feel-good neurochemicals of happiness, including:

- **Dopamine** (involved with anticipation, pleasure, and love)
- **Oxytocin** (involved with bonding and trust)
- **Endorphins** (involved with pain relief)

Singing along to a song can increase your levels of oxytocin too. Plus, when you sing it helps you take bigger breaths which can also help you be happy.

What types of music boost happiness?

- **Upbeat tunes** can distract you from pain and fatigue, while elevating your mood, and increasing your endurance.
- **Fast beats** tend to speed up your brain waves.
- **Relaxing music** can soothe your soul and lower cortisol, the stress hormone.
- **Classical** - Just 25 minutes of listening to Mozart or Strauss has been shown to lower stress (and blood pressure).
- **Calming music** is known to boost pleasurable feelings, improve mood, and help with focus and concentration, largely because it can increase dopamine levels.
- **Lullabies** and soothing music can help improve your sleep.

All of us have different preferences for music, depending on our brain type, age, and personality. Sometimes you may need calming music to induce pleasant feelings, and other times you may prefer upbeat music to lift you up and energize you.

Today's exercise: Identify and write down 10 songs that make you feel happy and create a feel-good playlist you can listen to for a mood boost.

"Music produces a kind of pleasure that human nature cannot do without."
— Confucius, The Book of Rites

DAY 24. LAUGH MORE
(Relates to Secret 2, 5, and 6)

So many people who took our 30-Day Happiness Challenge online have told me that this day's lesson is one of their favorites. Think of it as permission to let go, to feel like a kid again, and to have fun. It's all about laughter, something that has so many benefits for your brain. Being able to laugh—and laugh often—is a key component to boosting your happiness. Unfortunately, laughter seems to be in short supply, especially the older we become. Research found that the frequency with which we laugh or smile each day starts to plummet around age 23.

- Adults laugh an average of 4.2 times a day.
- Children laugh an average of 300 times a day!

It's time to change this, especially if you want to be happier. Every time you let out a chuckle, your brain releases the chemicals of happiness— dopamine, oxytocin, and endorphins. Laughing also lowers the stress hormone cortisol and can elevate your pain threshold. A healthy and hearty laugh is like a drug, changing your brain chemistry to make you feel happier, and making it happen almost instantly!

One of the best things about laughter is how good it is for you:

- It's contagious (the kind of contagion you want).
- Laughing together with others creates a bond.
- When you crack a joke and make someone else laugh, your brain releases a cocktail of feel-good neurochemicals that make you feel happy too.

Laughter truly is the best medicine!

Today's exercise: *Watch a comedy—a television series, a movie, or a stand-up comedy routine. For even more bonding, watch with someone you love.*

> *"Humor is mankind's greatest blessing."*
> *— Mark Twain*

DAY 25. RELATING
(Relates to Secret 6)

The people in your life can either fuel happiness or make you feel miserable. One of the most overlooked reasons why relationships either work well or fall apart is based on Brain Types. Understanding your Brain Type and the Brain Types of the people you love can help you navigate your way to happier relationships. The acronym, RELATING, can help you to remember the foundational relationship habits that optimize your chance of success.

R is for Responsibility: Taking responsibility for your role in your relationships helps you avoid the blame game. Conversely, pretending you are helpless gives your partner control over the relationship and fuels distress, anxiety, depression, resentment, and hopelessness.

E is for Empathy: Empathy helps you understand one another and is essential in relationships. Practice seeing things from the other person's point of view and learn what makes them happy or unhappy.

L is for Listening: Good communication is necessary for a strong relationship. You can improve your interpersonal communication by actively listening without interrupting.

A is for Assertiveness: Being assertive means expressing your thoughts and feelings in a firm yet reasonable way: not allowing others to emotionally run over you; and, not saying "yes" when you mean "no."

T is for Time: For healthy relationships, you must invest in "special time," when you can be present and focus on each other without distractions. Spend time doing things you both enjoy.

I is for Inquiry: People can get wrapped up in negative thinking patterns that sabotage their relationships. Whenever you have a distressing thought about yours, write it down and ask yourself if it's really true. Sometimes our thoughts lie to us!

N is for Noticing What You Like a Lot More than What You Don't Like: This practice, which is Secret 6, is called positive reinforcement—and it works!

G is for Grace: Grace and forgiveness play an instrumental role in helping relationships flourish—and can be powerfully healing.

Today's exercise: *Choose one letter from RELATING and practice that skill today.*

"Positive connections make us feel loved, secure, and content, while troubled relationships drive anxiety, stress, and unhappiness."
— Daniel G. Amen, MD

DAY 26. HAPPY SCENTS
(Relates to Secret 2)

Just like music (Day 23) can put you in a better mood, so can certain scents. The olfactory system in your brain—which gives you the ability to smell—is connected to your emotional centers. It's our oldest sense and because of that it can be very powerful in how you feel.

- Certain scents can trigger happiness for you. Often, they are connected to happy memories, and some scents in the natural world make us feel happy too.
- At the same time, certain scents can actually trigger anxiety and trauma if they're linked to bad memories from the past.
- It's also known that when the hippocampus deteriorates (it's close to the olfactory area of the brain), it's one of the predictors for Alzheimer's disease.

Some scents, like those found in essential oils, can boost your happiness by inducing a sense of calm, rejuvenation, and inspiration. Here are some of our favorites:

- Lavender can help reduce worries and depression and make you feel more relaxed
- Eucalyptus is revitalizing
- Jasmine is uplifting
- Peppermint is energizing
- Ylang Ylang helps reduce stress
- Chamomile is soothing
- Certain citrus smells can boost your mood and sharpen your focus

Spending time each day giving your nose a workout with scents that make you feel good can really help your level of happiness.

Today's exercise: *Identify the scents that make you happy.*

"Who doesn't need a reminder to smell the roses as we rush through life?"
— Daniel G. Amen, MD

DAY 27. ADOPT BRAIN-HEALTHY FOOD ROUTINES *(Relates to Secret 4)*

By now in your journey, you're probably realizing that creating and sticking to happiness habits are major components of becoming a happier person. Developing healthy routines and family traditions around food is a major part of the equation. You need to ask yourself if your food routines are helping you or hurting you. So often, people are stuck in their unhealthy habits, convincing themselves that they cannot give them up.

Saying something like, "I could never give up Rocky Road ice cream (or doughnuts, pasta, etc.)" is actually an ANT that's stuck in your head. Ask yourself the 5 questions to challenge that thought, and you'll recognize how invalid it is.

There are much healthier ways to enjoy treats, and they can be just as tasty and satisfying! For example, here are a couple of the ones my family enjoys regularly:

Decaf Cappuccino
- Unsweetened organic vanilla almond milk
- Decaf coffee (amount to your liking)
- Heat up the decaf and almond milk and add a couple spritzes of chocolate, vanilla, or pumpkin spice stevia from Sweet Leaf.
- Pour into a blender, put the lid on, and froth.
- Pour into your coffee mug and sprinkle with a combo of erythritol mixed with cinnamon.

Brain-Healthy Hot Chocolate
- Unsweetened organic vanilla almond milk
- Organic raw cacao (an amazing super food!)
- Heat up and add a few spritzes of chocolate stevia.
- It's less than 100 calories – and good for you!

Today's exercise: *Make some Brain-Healthy Hot Chocolate or a Decaf Cappuccino*

"Choose happy foods that make you feel better, not just for the moment but for the long run."— Daniel G. Amen, MD

DAY 28. ACTIVE LISTENING
(Relates to Secret 6)

On this day of your happiness journey, you're going to focus more closely on one of the RELATING skills you learned on Day 25: L is for Listening.

In particular, think about active listening. When you actively listen to other people, you strengthen the connection and increase the influence you have with them. Hearing others and feeling heard are important for having healthy relationships with friends, loved ones, and coworkers. Good communication is an essential component of any relationship, but not everyone is very good at it. By learning and practicing these 7 active listening skills, you can strengthen your connection, understanding, and sense of trust with others.

1. Decrease distractions (i.e. put down your phone).

2. Be present. Smile, nod silently, lean in, or say "I see," "I understand," "Uh-huh," or "Hmmm."

3. Make eye contact.

4. Don't interrupt. Sometimes people are worried that they are going to forget what they want to say, so they interrupt. But when that happens the person speaking can lose their train of thought, and the conversation goes in a completely different direction.

5. Don't judge, because when you do, it stops the conversation or leads to an argument.

6. Give the person some space and allow for periods of silence rather than filling up every second. Be patient and let them take their time.

7. Repeat back what has been said and listen for the feelings behind the words. When you are dismissive about what a person is saying, you diminish their feelings.

Today's exercise: *Practice Active Listening with your partner, child, or coworker. In the space below, write about how it went and how it made you feel.*

____

____

____

"Listening is a magnetic and strange thing, a creative force. The friends who listen to us are the ones we move toward. When we are listened to, it creates us, makes us unfold and expand." — Psychiatrist Karl A. Menninger

DAY 29. DIAPHRAGMATIC BREATHING
(Relates to Secrets 2 and 5)

Now that you're almost to the end of this 30-day journey, it's time to take a breath... literally! Breathing is so important because your brain is 2% of your body's weight, but it uses 20% of the oxygen you breathe. Being in any state of oxygen debt damages the brain, which is why holding your breath or sleep apnea are so bad for brain function.

You have two lungs in your chest, and between your chest and your belly, you have a bell-shaped muscle called the diaphragm. If you ever watch a baby or a puppy breathe, they breathe almost exclusively with their belly, which means when they breathe in, their diaphragm flattens, and their belly goes out. When they exhale, their diaphragm comes up, pushing air out.

Research has shown that if you take twice as long to breathe out than you do to breathe in, it triggers the opposite of a fight or flight response. This simple breathing pattern helps to reset your whole body which helps you feel better.

Diaphragmatic breathing is really simple. This exercise takes 3 minutes:

- **Inhale to a count of 3 - 4**
- **Exhale to a count of 6 - 8**
- **Repeat this pattern 10 times.**

If you need to practice breathing with your diaphragm instead of your chest, try this. Put one hand on your chest and one on your belly. Notice how you're breathing right now. If you're breathing with your chest, try this instead:

- Lie on your back and place a small book on your belly.
- When you breathe in, make the book go up, and when you breathe out, make the book go down.

Today's exercise: *Download the Awesome Breathing App and practice breathing deeply.*

"Don't forget to breathe." — Daniel G. Amen, MD

DAY 30. HAVE A BRAIN HEALTHY PARTY
(Relates to Secrets 1-7)

Congratulations on completing your 30-day happiness journey! It's time to celebrate in ways that support your ongoing happiness. You deserve to have a party, and there are so many fun and brain-healthy ways to do it. Be sure to invite people who lift you up, not those who bring you down.

Here are a few suggestions for how you can get that Happy Party rolling.

- Serve brain-healthy foods from the Happy Foods list in Day 5.
- Don't diminish your happiness by serving alcohol! Choose flavored seltzer, ice water with slices of fruit, or flavored stevia instead.
- Play music from the Happy Playlist you created on Day XX.
- Dance! It's fun and boosts your happy brain chemicals.
- Have a table tennis tournament—it will boost your brain's cerebellum.
- Write appreciation notes to each other and read them out loud.
- Watch a funny movie together.

How to Have a Brain-Healthy Party

Hosting a party with brain healthy fare is easy. Packed with potent antioxidants and nutrients, these party foods will boost brain function for a memorable and memory-enhancing soirée.

Holiday Spiced Green Tea
Mix green tea leaves with chopped and dried orange peel, chopped and dried ginger root, and cinnamon. Add unsweetened almond milk for a healthy version of a chai tea.

Spa Water
Serve sparkling or flat water with lemon or lime wedges.

Raw Veggies Tray
Broccoli florets
Red, yellow, orange, and green bell peppers
Cherry tomatoes
Carrots

Fruit Bowl
Fill a bowl with cherries.

Cheese Tray
Pair low-fat cheese with fruit like apples.

Hummus
Made from garbanzo beans, lemon juice, tahini, olive oil, and garlic.

Guacamole
Mix avocado with onions, tomatoes, serrano chiles, and lime or lemon juice.

Salsa
Combine tomatoes, onions, cilantro, jalapeno peppers, lime, garlic powder, and cumin.

Black Bean Dip
Purée low-salt or no-salt canned black beans, red onion, orange or lime juice, cilantro, olive oil, garlic, and cumin (found in curry) in a blender.

Mixed Nuts
Walnuts, almonds, cashews, and peanuts.

Bruschetta
Use gluten-free bread or crackers and top with heirloom tomatoes, a little olive oil, and lots of fresh basil.

Smoked Wild Salmon
Serve smoked wild salmon with lemon, capers, and dill on gluten-free toast points.

Pizza
Use gluten-free dough to make a thin crust, sprinkle lightly with low-fat cheese, top with oregano, and add grilled turkey or veggies like spinach, asparagus, and fresh tomato.

Chicken Skewers
Grill chicken breasts marinated in plain yogurt, curry, fresh ginger, and garlic.

Shrimp Kebabs
Marinate shrimp in olive oil, garlic, and lemon.

Shrimp Cocktail
Serve jumbo shrimp with homemade cocktail sauce made with low-sugar ketchup, horseradish, and lemon juice.

Sushi
Wrap sushi-grade wild salmon or tuna, avocado, cucumber, and asparagus in just a little brown rice then wrap with seaweed.

Edamame
Cooked soybeans go great with sushi.

Yogurt Parfait
Top plain Greek yogurt with blueberries, strawberries, and raspberries, then sprinkle with chopped almonds for a tasty dessert.

Today's exercise: *Retake the Oxford Happiness Questionnaire to see how your happiness score has changed.*

"Happiness doesn't just happen. You have to work at it every day. Keep working on it."
— Daniel G. Amen, MD

RESOURCES

AMEN CLINICS
www.amenclinics.com
888-288-9834

Locations:

ATLANTA
5901 Peachtree-Dunwoody Road, Suite C65
Atlanta, GA 30328

CHICAGO
2333 Waukegan, Suite 150
Bannockburn, IL 60015

DALLAS
7301 State Highway 161, Suite 170
Irving, TX 75039

LOS ANGELES
5363 Balboa Blvd., Suite 100
Encino, CA 91316

NEW YORK
16 E. 40th Street, 9th Floor
New York, NY 10016

ORANGE COUNTY, CA
3150 Bristol Street, Suite 400
Costa Mesa, CA 92626

SAN FRANCISCO
350 N. Wiget Lane, Suite 105
Walnut Creek, CA 94598

SEATTLE
616 120th Ave NE, Suite C100
Bellevue, WA 98005

SOUTH FLORIDA
200 South Park Road, Suite 140
Hollywood, FL 33021

WASHINGTON, D.C.
10701 Parkridge Blvd., Suite 110
Reston, VA 20191

BrainMD (high-quality supplements and brain health products)
wwww.BrainMD.com
High-quality, smarter supplements and
brain health products to optimize your
brain and your life.

Amen University
www.AmenUniversity.com
Master your health, emotions,
relationships, and more through
our library of easy-to-follow online
brain health courses to create a
brighter future.